Bike Shorts:

Your complete guide to indoor cycling

By Marisa Michael, RDN, LD, CPT

About the author

Marisa Michael, RDN, LD, CPT is a registered dietitian, personal trainer, and group exercise instructor. She specializes in sports nutrition and weight management. She absolutely loves cycling, indoors and out. She once got hit by a truck while riding her brand new road bike, and she *still* loves cycling.

Marisa stays in shape by cycling, teaching exercise classes, swimming, and running. Well, "running" is a strong word; it's more like a slow jog.

Marisa has completed several triathlons, ranging from sprint distance (12 miles) to half-iron distance (70.3 miles). She once swam from San Francisco to Alcatraz without getting eaten by sharks. She has eaten unknown gallons of ice cream (maybe she should have kept track?) and appreciates every bite.

She has three children whom she once convinced to do a triathlon. Results were mixed. Her husband is not nearly so gullible and hasn't done a single triathlon. Yet.

Her qualifications include Registered Dietitian Nutritionist, Licensed Dietitian, Certified Personal Trainer, Certified Group Exercise Instructor, Certificate of Training in Weight Management, Certified Indoor Cycle Instructor by Mad Dogg Indoor Cycling (Spinning brand), Keiser M3 Indoor Cycling, and the International Olympic Committee's Diploma in Sports Nutrition.

Marisa owns a private dietetic practice, and also teaches exercise and nutrition classes at a local health club. She lives in Oregon, USA.

Table of Contents

Bike Shorts: Chapter 1

Introduction

You're at your local gym, minding your own business. Maybe doing a few crunches, or trying out that new piece of equipment. When all of a sudden you hear it: the *thwump thwump thwump* of the speakers from the cycle studio. Why does it always sound like they're playing either synthesizer music from the 90's, or unintelligible rap? Why does everyone shuffle out of there dripping in sweat, as if they have been hosed down? And *why is it always so packed?*

You decide there must be something amazing about this indoor cycling thing, because everybody who's anyone is doing it. Your neighbor swears it helped her lose her maternity weight. Your type A financial advisor claims it's a great stress reliever. You're reluctantly convinced that you should probably venture into one of those cycle classes and see what it's all about.

The problem is, where do you start? It can be intimidating. You heard something about special shoes? And a bike fit? Everyone always looks so beat after class. And can you bring yourself to wear those *shorts?*

If you are a seasoned indoor cyclist, but stopped going, it is time to rediscover your love for cycling. Maybe you couldn't figure out how to rehydrate and got a headache every single time. Maybe your bike wasn't set up right and soreness got the best of you. Whatever the reason, it's time to get back in the saddle.

Whether you are a novice or an expert, there's something for everyone in this book. *Bike Shorts* is a series of short chapters (or "shorts") on anything you might need to know about indoor cycling. Each "short" will cover a different topic. You can read straight through, or you can just go to the chapter that suits your needs.

"Shorts" topics include:

- Why cycle? Health benefits and more
- What to expect at your first class
- Cycling etiquette
- Suggested gear: the scoop on shoes and other essentials
- Developing technique and form
- Types of bikes and classes
- Nutrition and hydration for before, during, and after a session
- Workout plans for you to do on your own

Settle in for a good read to help you have a great ride.

Bike Shorts: Chapter 2

Why indoor cycling?

Cycling inside may sound boring. Comedian Jim Gaffigan jokes in his *Mr. Universe* show that a stationary bike is a "bike that goes nowhere." While it's true you can't explore the countryside with your gym's Spinning® bike, there are some real benefits to indoor cycling.

Many people love the camaraderie that accompanies a cycle class. There is something invigorating about having a room full of people who are all trying to sprint as hard as they can together, ride that tough hill together, and enjoy the cool down together. Friendships are strengthened along with cardiovascular fitness.

An indoor cycle class, believe it or not, can offer variety beyond an outdoor cycle session. Through use of music, intervals, speed, and resistance, a talented instructor can craft a different class every time.

For those seasoned road cyclists that have seen all sorts of dangerous conditions, from rain, snow, wind, potholes, darkness, to inattentive drivers, indoor cycling can offer a safe way to enjoy cycling as a sport without the hazards of outdoor cycling.

Athletes that are looking for a specific training regimen can better achieve it indoors. Where can you find terrain that allows you to climb a hill for exactly 30 seconds, then sprint on a flat for exactly 30 seconds, and do that for five repeats? Indoor sessions can offer precision unmatched in the outdoor world for specific training goals.

Those with knee or hip injuries often find solace in the cycle studio. Often a runner who has been sidelined with an injury can still cycle without pain, making it a great way to maintain fitness while injured.

There are real and proven health benefits to cycling. As with most exercise, health benefits can include improved cardiovascular function, decreased risk of chronic disease, increased lean muscle mass, increased joint mobility, decreased body fat, better weight management, stress relief, reduced risk of premature death, and improved mood and mental health.[1] Cycling in particular also offers a low-impact sport for those with joint issues, poor bone health, or gait and mobility issues.

Now that you are totally convinced that indoor cycling is for you (except maybe the Spandex), keep reading for what to expect at your first class.

Bike Shorts: Chapter 3

What to expect at your first class

If you are a newbie to the cycle world, this "short" is the most important one. If you are experienced but want to brush up, keep reading—you may pick up a few tips and tricks you hadn't known about before.

First, be sure to come early. Often instructors are there 10-15 minutes before class starts to set up their music and to help newcomers like you. Approach the instructor and introduce yourself, explaining that you've never done this before and you need a bike fit. The instructor will help get you set up properly.

There is a science to getting the correct fit. The instructor should pay attention to saddle (seat) height, how your knees line up with the pedal, and the angle of your hips, elbows, and shoulders. Different brands of bikes adjust differently: some have fore and aft adjustments on the handlebars, some don't. All bikes have adjustable saddle height, fore and aft saddle position, and handlebar height.

A correct fit should feel like this:

Hands lie gently on the handlebars; shoulders are not rounded forward. Elbows are soft, meaning you don't have to extend your reach just to grasp the handlebars. Your shoulders are back and chest is open. Your back is flat with a nice neutral curve in the lower back. You are hinged at the hip to leverage your quadriceps muscles, which are your thighs or the top of the upper leg.

When you pedal, your knees are lined up with the middle of your shoelaces or the pedal spindle (where the pedal connects to the crank arm). Knees are lined up, not bowing in or splayed out. They feel like they could drive upward and line up with your chest, although they won't physically touch that high.

Your saddle is high enough to get a soft bend in the knee, but not so high that when your foot is closest to the ground you would have to rock your hip to reach down, or lock out your knee. When your foot is in the pedal and closest to the ground, your knee should have a soft bend. Experts recommend 15-37° knee bend.

Your buttocks are back on the widest part of the saddle, not forward toward the nose of the saddle. Your feet are secured in the pedal either by a cycling shoe cleat or a toe cage—more on that later. Heels are dropped down and ankles are relaxed. You could wiggle your toes in your shoe and feel the ball of your foot on the pedal.

If you are wearing cycling shoes, you should be clipped into the pedal and feel connected to it. If you are wearing athletic shoes and utilizing the toe cage, cinch the straps up around your shoe so it feels snug. This will enable you to get a more powerful, efficient pedal stroke.

It should feel comfortable to spin at an easy tempo with a little resistance. Resistance is the friction placed on the bike's flywheel to mimic the feeling of a road under a real bike tire. There needs to be some resistance at all times, just like on a real bike. If you pedal with no resistance, you will end up bouncing in your seat, damaging your knees, and wasting a workout that could have been useful in building your fitness.

Your instructor can orient you to the bike's features. You need to know how to add resistance in order to ride the bike. Many bikes have a knob to turn that increases resistance as you turn it clockwise (the Keiser brand bikes have levers that increase resistance). The knob is also an emergency brake. If you feel out of control with the pedal stroke, push down directly on the knob. This will slow and stop the flywheel and pedals.

If your cycle studio has bikes with computer consoles, ask the instructor to explain how to use it and what the numbers mean.

Common data displayed on the console include:

Revolutions per minute (rpms): This is also referred to as cadence. It is the speed at which you are pedaling. 60-80 rpms is considered a "hill," and 80-110 rpms is considered a "flat." 110 rpms is an all-out sprint. The instructor will often give a goal rpm to achieve. For instance, the instructor might say, "We are going to do a flat road at an endurance pace for 60 seconds, so get to 90 rpms." Or "Let's sprint! I want to see 110 rpms all out! Go! go! go!" At which point you speed up like a hamster on a wheel and hope the rest of the class doesn't notice how hard you are wheezing.

Time: It will usually display the total time you have been riding. Yup, that's it.

Heart rate: Some bikes are designed to sync with your own personal heart rate monitor (if you are wearing one — more on that in the "gear" section).

Distance: The bike estimates distance based on the speed and time you have been riding. This is usually a little inaccurate, so don't get too excited when you see you've gone 20 miles in 35 minutes.

Calories burned: Some bikes display your estimated calories burned, usually based on your speed and time riding. The calories burned is usually very inaccurate because the bike computer doesn't know your gender, height, weight, age, or body composition, all of which are crucial to know actual calories burned. While it's cool to see that you torched some calories during your session, don't get too hung up on the numbers. If you need more specifics for your particular bike, ask the instructor to clarify how the bike calculates how many calories you burned.

Watts: This is the power output you generate while riding. Watts is a function of force and speed. If you are cycling with heavy tension and also going fast, you will generate more watts (power) than if you are cycling at lighter tension and slower pace. If you can generate higher watts with less effort, it means you are in better shape. What's cool about watts is that you can see fitness gains over time. If, when you started cycling, you could only average about 90 watts per class, but a few months later you can do 110 watts per class and it doesn't feel any harder, you know you've made fitness gains. Cyclists love to geek out on the numbers, and experienced cyclists love using their watts output to achieve specific training outcomes. In general, you should be able see an average wattage reading for your session that is roughly equal to your weight. For example, if you weigh 160 pounds, you should be able to average 160 watts per class. If you regularly average more, great job! You are a beast!

The class format will vary based on the instructor and the type of gym you go to. But most have some commonalities which you can expect.

Indoor cycling attempts to duplicate on some level what you might find on an outdoor ride. That means some "flat" roads with less resistance, some "hills" with more resistance, and some standing up out of the saddle. When you stand, be sure to add more resistance (by turning a knob or pushing a lever, depending on the type of bike) to compensate for the increased gravity you are now placing on the pedals. Too little resistance when you stand means trouble for your knees and your workout. You'll have to tweak it until you find what feels right to you.

A class not only has "flats" and "hills," but also utilizes different speeds. An endurance speed feels like a steady pace, where you are breathing somewhat hard, but it is sustainable. Usually this is around 80-100 rpms. Intervals are short sets (usually less than 60 seconds) of very hard work, such as a flat sprint or a steep hill. They are designed to build fitness in a specific way, and always need to be accompanied by recovery (pedaling slowly with light resistance). Sprints are around 110 rpms. If you are sprinting, but going over 120 rpms, it's time to add some resistance.

The instructor usually designs the class in such a way to give some variety. Often a ride corresponds with the beat of the music. For instance, if the instructor is playing an upbeat song with a strong chorus, the sprint portion of the workout might come during the chorus. Allow the music to inspire you to ride better, faster, and stronger. Dynamic music can push you harder than you would have on your own. This results in a fun and satisfying workout.

Take note: you don't always have to follow the instructor. If you feel like it is too steep, too fast, or too hard, back off on the speed or the resistance. Especially for your first few classes, don't feel like you must keep up with the class. The beauty of indoor cycling is that people of all different fitness levels can ride together and enjoy the synergy that comes with a unified class. Many people turn the resistance knob down or slow their pedal speed when they are unable to perform what the instructor is demanding. This enables them to still complete the class and work at their own pace. Some others may go harder or faster than the instructor prompts. This is also ok—these people may need to achieve a specific athletic or training goal. You can customize your workout for how you are feeling that day.

While it's a good idea to keep up with the class as much as you can (otherwise, why are you there?), don't feel undue pressure to perform in a way you're not physically ready for yet. Most instructors know this and are happy to accommodate all levels. If you are getting the vibe that you need to keep up when you are not ready to, try a different instructor.

The overall class should look like this:

- Come early to get set up, about 10-15 minutes beforehand.
- Warm up, 5-10 minutes, following instructor cues.
- Workout portion, which could include endurance riding, hills, sprints, or technique drills.
- Cool down, 5-10 minutes.
- Stretch.
- Clean off bike and stumble to your car, satisfied you got a killer workout.

Now you know what to expect and how to set up your bike. It's time to learn about a few etiquette guidelines. Read on!

Bike Shorts: Chapter 4

Cycling Etiquette and Tips

Cyclists can sometimes be a quirky bunch. This is especially true for some experienced athletes who have been riding for years and have become set in their ways.

Knowing some basic etiquette can save you some embarrassment and help maximize your workout.

Don't use your phone during class. The instructor has created a playlist and ride profile just for your class. It's inconsiderate to be on your phone, text, browse social media, read an e-book (except maybe this one...) or ride with your own headphones and music. If you are doing these things, you don't need a class. Just ride on your own. Many classes take place in dim lighting to promote focus and minimize distractions. A bright phone screen will detract from the atmosphere of the class. Be respectful to the instructor and your classmates and engage fully in the ride.

Minimize chatting with your neighbor. Cycling is a great for building friendships, but keep the chatting contained to the beginning of class when everyone is setting up and warming up, before the instructor officially starts. Chatting is distracting to those around you. And if you are chatting, are you really working as hard as you could be?

Keep your stuff contained. It's really easy to crowd a cycle studio with lots of workout bags and gear, but this can create trip hazards and a less-than-Zen environment. Try corralling your belongings by leaving them in your car, locker, or a cubby.

Come ready to engage. If you are only half-committed, you won't get the workout you crave and it will detract from the rest of class. Be ready and willing to give it your all.

Let the instructor know if you need to leave early. Imagine being an instructor: you put your heart, time, and probably your own money into the perfect playlist. You planned an interesting and effective workout. If someone gets up and leaves, the instructor wonders, "Why?" Did they not like the song? Is it too loud? Is the class too hard? Too easy? Is it too hot in here? Is the bike not working properly? Are they about to pass out? Do they need medical attention? Letting the instructor know ahead of time that you need to leave early is common courtesy and saves worry.

Clean the bike and your area after class. Sweat is going to happen. Some people leave literal puddles of it on the floor. Most gyms provide sanitizing wipes to clean off the bikes after class (if your gym doesn't have this, ewww! Switch gyms!). Wipe the saddle, handlebars, resistance knob, and anything else you got sweaty. Avoid wiping the computer, as the moisture can damage it. You can use a towel to wipe the floor.

Ok, so now you know some basic cycling manners. Now it's time to find out if you really need to wear tight Lycra bike shorts. It's all about gear in the next chapter.

Bike Shorts: Chapter 5

All about cycling gear. Or, "Do these bike shorts make me look fat?"

The fitness industry is chock full of people trying to sell you things. Cycling in particular seems to offer an array of products you wouldn't ever know you needed. Compression socks anyone? How about $150 padded bike shorts? Or maybe you need that $25 water bottle with the fancy filter? Do you need a wearable tracking device, like FitBit? Or a heart rate monitor? You can quickly spend hundreds of dollars in cycling gear, but you may not need it all.

Here are some suggestions for gear essentials.

Buy the shoes. Really, do it. But only after you've done classes for a month and know that you are really going to stick with it. If you are even a casual indoor cyclist, popping in every week or two, you need the shoes. Expect to spend $100-300. Cycling shoes are specially designed to be incredibly stiff. They support your foot and help you get a better pedal stroke. They prevent injury. And they last a long, long time. It's worth the investment.

A cleat is a metal clip that screws into the bottom of a cycle shoe, and clicks into the pedal on the bike. Check with your gym to see what kind of cleat you need. Most use SPD or LOOK Delta cleats. A friendly bike shop salesperson will help you select shoes and cleats, and they often install the cleats for you as well. If you install your own cleats, make sure you screw them on tightly. Place them where they line up with the ball of your foot.

Mountain bike shoes are best for indoor cycling. They are designed with thick outsoles around the cleat area, which protects the cleat while you walk on the ground. Road bike shoes are designed with flat soles, and the metal cleat protrudes out, making it difficult to walk without hitting the cleat on the ground.

To attach your shoe/cleat system to the bike pedal, first get on the bike. Put one shoe on the pedal, making sure the pedal is flipped to the side that will accept cleats. Place the cleat toe- side in first, then drop your heel down until you feel it click into place. An instructor can help you if you can't figure out how to clip in. It should feel comfortable with your toes pointed forward and knees lined up with the pedal spindle (where the pedal attaches to the crank arm). To detach from the pedal, simply rotate your heel outward (away from the bike) and the pedal clip will disengage from the cleat.

There is a phenomenon called "float," which means that, when you are clipped into the pedal, you should be able to move your shoe side to side a tiny bit. The cleat should feel like it is "floating" in the pedal clip. This allows for movement within the pedal stroke that is not so restrictive that it will lead to injury.

If you try out your shiny new shoes and feel discomfort, numbness, or tingling in your feet, adjust the cleats and re-check your bike fit. Bikefit.com has excellent guidelines with illustrations for fine-tuning your bike fitting needs. If discomfort persists even with tweaking your bike fit, there is something about the foot/pedal interface that is irritating your foot. If possible, try a different brand of shoe or cleat/pedal system.

Buy the shorts. But only if you have a sore bum after a month or so of cycling. Most people get used to the saddle and don't need any padding, but many people really like the padding that cycle shorts provide. They won't make you look fat, I promise. Well, maybe they'll give you sausage legs. Just own it. It's a great look. Another option is to buy a seat cover that you can place on the saddle each time you ride. They are squishy and hook right on top of the saddle.

Wear appropriate clothing. Athletic clothing with technical fabric that wicks away sweat will help you feel more cool and comfortable during the ride. Don't wear baggy or flared pants, because they can get caught in the crank arm or flywheel. Not only is that unsafe, it's just plain embarrassing. The right clothing will set you up for a great ride. And you'll look oh-so-stylish.

Bring a towel. If your studio doesn't provide towels, you will want to bring your own. Unlike outdoor cycling, where the natural wind cools your sweat, indoor studios can be stifling with minimal air movement. A towel is a lifesaver for wiping sweat dripping into your eyes. And believe me, you will sweat!

Heart rate monitors are optional. They can be really, really useful for specific training goals and more effective training. But if you are a casual rider or don't want to spend the extra money, you can certainly build fitness without one. Before you purchase, check with your gym to see if their bikes sync with certain brands of heart rate monitors. Some bike computer consoles can wirelessly display the data from your heart rate monitor strap.

If you decide to use a heart rate monitor, you need to know what the numbers mean. Here is a short run-down.

There are a lot of different formulas to estimate maximum heart rate and heart rate work zones. A common formula to find maximum heart rate is:

Males: 220-age=maximum heart rate.

Females: 226-age=maximum heart rate.

For example, if you are a 40-year-old male, 220-40=180 beats per minute (bpm) is your maximum heart rate.

Next, use this maximum heart rate to determine different training zones.

Training zones/heart rate zones vary based on which manual you consult, but here are some general heart rate zones:

Easy/Recovery zone: 50-65% of maximum heart rate

Moderate/Endurance zone: 65-75% of maximum heart rate

Hard/Threshold: 75-85% of maximum heart rate

Very hard/Anaerobic: 85-95% of maximum heart rate

So using the above example of a 40-year-old male with 180 bpm maximum heart rate, you then calculate how many beats per minute would fall into each zone.

Here's what it looks like:

Easy/Recovery zone: 50-65% of maximum means 180 bpm x .5 (or 50%)=90 bpm and 180 bpm x .65 (or 65%)=117 bpm. So if you are a 40-year old male and want to work out in a recovery or easy zone, you would pedal until your heart rate monitor displayed between 90-117 bpm.

Moderate/Endurance zone: 65-75% of maximum is 117-135 bpm.

Hard/Threshold: 75-85% of maximum is 135-153 bpm.

Very hard/Anaerobic: 85-95% of maximum is 153-171 bpm.

All sorts of athletes, from recreational to professional, use heart rate zones for specific training goals. Your instructor might cue you to get to an "anaerobic" zone on a sprint. If you have a heart rate monitor, you'll know to get up to 153-171 bpm. It's a precise way to train and build fitness.

A word about heart rate: it can vary based on a lot of different factors. If it is especially hot or humid, if you are sick, stressed, overtrained, at high altitude, or taking certain medications, your heart rate might be higher than normal. There is also a lag time between what your heart is actually doing and what the monitor is reflecting.

In addition, a phenomenon called cardiovascular drift can occur. This is when your heart rate "drifts" higher within a workout, even when you haven't increased intensity. This may happen if your core temperature is too hot or you are in a humid environment. A heart rate monitor can let you know that your heart is pumping disproportionately high for the actual workload you are doing. Take note and drink sufficient fluids and reduce your work load as necessary.

If you don't have a heart rate monitor, but still want to judge which zone you may be working out in, there is something called the Rate of Perceived Exertion, or RPE scale.

The most common scale is the Modified Borg Scale for RPE. It looks like this:

0: No exertion

1: Very easy

2: Easy

3: Moderate

4: Somewhat hard

5-6: Hard

7-9: Very Hard

10: Maximal exertion

When you ride without a heart rate monitor, you can mentally check in with yourself every 5-10 minutes. Ask yourself, "On a scale of 0-10, how hard am I working?" If it's a 0-2: What the heck? Go harder! If it's a 4-8, that's probably just right. Adjust your workload to meet your fitness goals.

Now that you are a guru on gear, it is time to learn about technique and form.

Bike Shorts: Chapter 6

Technique and form

Good form enables you to have a comfortable, effective ride. It also helps prevent injury. Glance back to Chapter 1 where a correct bike fit is described. This is good form. Although it may seem simple to ride a stationary bike, there is a bit of technique to it that will help you succeed in your fitness goals. It will also help you get through the class!

Poor form or a poor bike setup can lead to your quadriceps muscles getting fatigued before they should, lower back pain, shoulder or wrist pain, and saddle soreness. A good bike fit can make a world of a difference in how enjoyable the class is and how effective your workout is.

Saddle soreness is normal for the first few classes, but it should go away as you get used to riding. If it persists, there are a few things you can do.

- First, double check your bike fit. This includes saddle height, fore/aft position, cleat position on your shoes (or shoe position on the pedal if you aren't using cycle shoes), handlebar height, and handlebar fore/aft position. Get a friendly instructor to help you figure out if anything looks wrong.
- If your bike fit is great, you can buy some padded cycle shorts. Many people like the extra comfort this provides.
- If you can't bring yourself to be seen in public in tight cycle shorts (seriously, it's not that embarrassing), you can purchase a padded cycle seat cover mentioned earlier. These can be found at any store that sells cycle gear. They are usually $15-25.

Your pedal stroke should feel smooth. Your feet should be spinning in smooth circles with no jerks, dead spots, or rebounding. Your ankle should feel neutral with your toes loose in your shoes. Don't point your toes downward during any part of the pedal stroke. Imagine you are powering a lightbulb with your bike. Keeping the pedal stroke smooth would ensure that the lightbulb doesn't flicker or fade, but rather is a steady source of light.

For perfecting technique, utilize mirrors in the cycle studio to observe yourself while you ride. You should look like your body is squared up to the bike, not leaning to one side or moving side to side. Your knees are lined up with the pedals. Your upper body feels relaxed with your shoulders down and a flat back. A loose grip on the handlebars and soft elbows will ensure a smooth cadence. You should feel like your elbows are tucked in a bit and you are having a strong forward movement. If you feel like you are bouncing in the saddle, add a little more tension with your resistance knob. You shouldn't have so little tension that your hips bounce or rock side to side. (Note: if hips rock, your saddle is probably too high).

Keeping your upper body relaxed will help to prevent fatigue. If you are tensing up muscles that aren't even used to propel the pedals, you are wasting energy that should be diverted to your legs. Remind yourself every so often to wiggle your toes, to drop your heels down, and to relax your shoulders, bringing them back and down. Keep your chest open. This will help you stay in good form to maximize efficiency and have an effective workout.

You might have been in a class where an instructor told you to "pull in your abs" or "tighten your core." This is actually incorrect. Good cycling form allows your midsection to be disengaged enough to support proper breathing. Tightening abdominals actually just flexes muscles that don't need to be flexed, which can divert energy away from your legs and into your upper body. This compromises breathing, form, and power.

Cycling does use core muscles to some extent, to maintain balance and form (and steering when outdoors). But a powerful and effective cyclist would never purposefully flex the abdominals while riding.

Many people wonder if cycling will make their legs bulk up. Women especially are sometimes worried that their quads will start to look like a speed skater over time. The answer is: no. Indoor cycling doesn't have enough resistance to build muscle in that fashion (called muscle hypertrophy). It will help you get leaner if you burn excess fat or calories while riding, but to get body-builder type legs you'd have to hit the weight room.

There are a few things you definitely should not do on the bike. Some instructors actually teach these things, but they are contraindicated. They use muscle groups in a potentially harmful manner. These can lead to injury at worst or an ineffective workout at best:

Pedaling backwards. Really, just don't do it. It does nothing good for your body, and usually it is harmful to the bike itself.

Doing pushups on the handlebars. I know, you just read that and thought, "What? How could I even *do* that?" I know, right? It makes no sense. Every nationally recognized cycle certification program tells instructors NEVER to do pushups on the bike. There are entire classes built around doing tiny "pushups" to the beat while spinning your feet wildly. Not only do you get an ineffective pushup, but your pedal stroke, quality, and intensity is compromised when you are trying to do a pushup. So you are simultaneously doing a poor pushup and a poor cycle workout. If you encounter one of these classes, steer clear. Your body deserves better.

Doing anything else other than cycling. And doing anything you wouldn't do on a bike while riding outside. This includes doing hand weights (save that for the weight room), stretching on the bike (especially while clipped into the pedals), leaning on your arms from side to side while doing tiny "pushups," and aiming shoulders and/or hips from side to side (called "tap-backs," often done while standing, spinning with little resistance at high speeds). Also no spinning with very little tension. This will set you up for a worthless workout and knee, tendon, or ligament injury. All these movements are contraindicated, meaning they will lead to injury and do not utilize muscle groups correctly.

Good technique can help you achieve a higher level of fitness and result in an effective and enjoyable ride. If you've forgotten everything you just read by the time you embark on your first cycle class, don't worry—just enjoy the ride and give it your best effort. A good instructor will cue with little prompts throughout the class, such as, "Loosen your upper body," or "Line up your knees with the pedal and smooth out your stroke." These cues will help you keep your form as you work out.

Keep reading for more intel on different types of bikes and class formats, so you can pick the one that works best for you.

Bike Shorts: Chapter 7

Types of bikes

There are a lot of different types of stationary bikes out there. This is a short list of some common ones you might find in a health club setting.

Direct contact resistance bikes: These bikes include Spinning brand, Schwinn, Technogym, LeMond, and others. These are the most common in indoor cycle studios. It's what you're probably picturing when you think of an indoor bike — chunky metal frame with a heavy flywheel (a metal disc about 40-50 pounds) and substantial handlebars. They feature a resistance knob. Resistance is created by the turning the knob, which pushes a felt pad (or other material) against the flywheel. It makes it harder to pedal, making it feel like you are climbing a hill. This is called direct-contact resistance.

Magnetic resistance bikes: These bikes are amazing. Keiser brand makes these bikes. If your gym has these, consider yourself blessed by the cycle gods. They are different from other bikes, in that the resistance is created by a magnetic flywheel. These bikes have precise gears and a very smooth ride. The computer not only displays the usual rpms, time, and distance, but it also has watts. This power output display is key to training effectively and building fitness. These bikes are the Porsche of the indoor cycling world.

Recumbent bikes: These are designed a little differently, so that you are sitting more upright or even a little back. The whole geometry is different from other indoor bikes. You won't find these in an indoor cycling studio. They are for a less intense ride and are sometimes used by people with lower back problems.

Fan-based resistance bikes: You might have seen these before—they look a little 1980's with a huge fan in front where it looks like a flywheel should be. They also have handlebars that move back and forth, like an elliptical. These are also not designed for a cycle class, but are in some gyms on the fitness floor. It is required to wear a sweatband and leg warmers while using this bike (just kidding).

Freewheel bikes: CycleOps manufactures unique bikes that are different from any other bike on the market. These freewheel bikes are not like a direct contact or magnetic resistance bike. Most bikes have a heavy flywheel in which the pedals and flywheel turn in sync. If the flywheel is turning, so do the pedals. This design flaw allows for a cyclist to "cheat": you can be pedaling with very little resistance and very little muscle recruitment, but the pedals are still turning and it looks like you are working. This means you could get an ineffective workout.

The freewheel design allows the wheel to turn independently from the pedals. As you turn the pedals, the freewheel will start spinning. It has a resistance knob and a pad that creates friction on the wheel, just like direct contact resistance bikes, but the difference is that the pedals do not continue to spin unless you are actually pedaling. This design forces you to use an efficient, full pedal stroke and a lot of leg muscle. It's a good bike that will give you a great workout.

Continue on to the next "short" for intel on class formats.

Bike Shorts: Chapter 8

Class formats

Endurance rides: Imagine you are riding outdoors for 25 miles or more. How fast would you go? You'd have a steady pace that you could maintain for a long time. This is an endurance ride. These are designed to be moderately hard with a tempo you can maintain for 30-60 minutes. You won't find intense sprints or steep hills in this format. This kind of ride is great for distance cycle training, triathlon training, or building a fitness base. This is conducted solely within an aerobic heard rate zone, around 65-75% of maximum heart rate and 80-100 rpms. RPE is about 4-7.

Hills: An skilled instructor wouldn't construct an entire class made of hills (there has to be some recovery for an effective workout), but you should count on a few hills in almost any indoor cycling class. A "hill" is created by adding more resistance, thereby slowing the flywheel and making it harder to pedal. It will feel like climbing a real hill outdoors. If the instructor cues you to stand (getting "out of the saddle"), make sure you have additional resistance to protect your knees. Keep your pedal stroke smooth and even, and avoid bouncing or rebounding on the pedals.

Hills can be in a moderate endurance zone, with an aerobic heart rate of 65-75%, or they can be a more intense, short interval at an anaerobic pace at 75-95% of maximum heart rate. A true "hill" in a cycle class encompasses the rpm range of about 60-80 rpms. If you are going faster than this, you could add more resistance. If you are going slower than this, you are opening yourself up for injury with too much torque on your knees.

Intervals: Intervals are short bursts of intense effort at an anaerobic heart rate. This could be created by a steep hill, "running" up a hill, sprinting up a hill, or sprinting on a flat road. Whatever the interval entails, it is all-out effort and for less than 60 seconds. Also called high-intensity interval training (or HIIT), this is a scientifically-proven and physiologically sound way to build cardiovascular fitness.

When you participate in interval training, you should feel very uncomfortable during the interval, with a high heart rate and heavy breathing. Heart rate zone is 65-95% of maximum heart rate, with rpms up to 110 for an all-out sprint. If you can exceed 120 rpms, put a little more resistance on to protect your knees and ligaments. RPE is around 9-10. Intervals are followed by a recovery period (about 30-120 seconds), before moving on to the next interval.

Strength ride: This is a ride designed to develop increased power output (measured in watts on a bike computer) and muscular endurance. This session would feel like an endurance ride, but with heavier resistance. Kind of like a really long, gradual hill. Usually the instructor would have the class both sit in the saddle and stand out of the saddle, mostly for comfort, but also to allow for different muscle recruitment. It is conducted in the heart rate zone around 75-85% of maximum heart rate. RPE is around 6-8.

Recovery ride: The name says it all. This is a relaxing, easy ride with normal resistance at 50-65% of maximum heart rate, and around 70-90 rpms. Recovery rides are useful after a tough workout the day before. An instructor may incorporate mental imagery and breathing exercises into this type of ride. RPE is around 3-5.

A little bit of everything: Most indoor cycle classes aren't dedicated to one particular format, but rather have a little bit of everything. This allows for interest and fun for participants. Expect to have some endurance sets, a couple hills, and a few sprints in any indoor cycle class. Be ready to try it, even if it seems daunting. You will thank yourself later!

Along with class formats, here's a list of some common exercises you might encounter in class. Read on, because it's nice to know the lingo. When the instructor shouts, "Ok, time for a pyramid!" you'll know exactly what to do. Don't get too worried about memorizing these. A good instructor will cue seamlessly, so you can mentally relax and focus on a productive, meaningful ride.

Ladders: This is a series of structured intervals and recoveries. The interval is the same amount of time as the recovery, building time as you go. For example, a sprint ladder would look like this:

1. Sprint 30 seconds, 110 rpms
2. Recover 30 seconds
3. Sprint 60 seconds, 110 rpms
4. Recover 60 seconds
5. Sprint 90 seconds, 110 rpms
6. Recover 90 seconds

See a pattern? You recover for the same time that you were sprinting and just go a little longer each time.

Pyramids: These are also structured interval and recoveries. But the recovery doesn't get longer with a longer interval, and you taper time up and down. A hill pyramid would look like this:

1. Climb 30 seconds, 60 rpms
2. Recover 30 seconds
3. Climb 60 seconds, 60 rpms
4. Recover 30 seconds
5. Climb 90 seconds, 60 rpms
6. Recover 30 seconds
7. Climb 120 seconds, 60 rpms
8. Recover 30 seconds
9. Climb 90 seconds, 60 rpms
10. Recover 30 seconds
11. Climb 60 seconds, 60 rpms
12. Recover 30 seconds
13. Climb 30 seconds, 60 rpms
14. Recover 30 seconds

Notice this pattern? All the recoveries are only 30 seconds. But each climb is shorter, then longer, then shorter again.

Sprints: These can be on a "flat" or on a "hill," depending on how much resistance you add. You accelerate up to 110 rpms. It feels tough, fast, and breathless. It's also really short, less than 60 seconds for a true sprint. Be sure not to let your butt bounce while you sprint. If this happens, add enough tension on your resistance knob to ensure that your hips do not rock or bounce, thereby protecting your knees and making an effective, powerful sprint.

Hill sprints: Just what it sounds like, sprinting up a hill. Fun! Heavy resistance creates a leg-burning, lung-searing burst of power with a skyrocketing heart rate. It's a great way to build aerobic fitness, but do it with proper form and recovery.

Jumps/lifts: Picture yourself riding on a steep hill outside. It's so steep you stand up to ride. But then your heart rate spikes too much and your pedaling isn't efficient. You get tired too quickly. So you sit down. Then your legs start to burn, and you think standing up might be easier. So you do the best of both: alternate sitting and standing every few pedal strokes. This is a jump, or lift, in a cycle class. Usually it is done to the beat of the music: every 8 beats, sit; the next 8 beats, stand; and so on. It's a strategy used in real-world outdoor cycling to get up a long, steep hill. Use caution when doing these: if you don't have enough resistance, it can hurt your knees. Don't do it if you can't keep good form, making sure to keep your body weight off the handlebars. You should feel muscle engagement in the gluteal (butt) and quadriceps (top of thigh) area. Don't be afraid to skip this move if you are not ready for it. It needs to be done properly to be safe and effective.

Intervals: This can be anything that is a short, intense, all-out effort. A hill, a sprint, a sprint on a hill, a run, a seated push — anything that is hard! This always needs to be accompanied by a recovery period.

Drills: Drills are designed to work a specific aspect of your cycling program. It may target pedal stroke efficiency, a heart rate zones, breathing, or anything else. There are a ton of different drills out there. Here are a few examples to try out.

  _ *Push/pull:* Staying seated, gradually add resistance until it feels steep enough that you would want to stand up (but stay seated!). Relax your upper body, shift your buttocks to the widest part of the saddle, keep your back flat and hinge at the hip. Focus your mind on how your feet feel in contact with the pedal. It should feel like the pedal is connected to the ball of your foot with even pressure all the way around the stroke, and your heels are dropped down. Concentrate on making your feet feel like they are going in smooth circles. Now shift how you pedal: think about the top part of the stroke, leading to the bottom (closest to the floor). If your feet were making a circle on a clock, the bottom is 6 o'clock and the top is 12 o'clock. From 12 o'clock to 6 o'clock, push down a little harder, trying to generate extra power. After a minute or two, shift how you pedal again: this time think about the backstroke, from 6 o'clock at the bottom back up to 12 o'clock. It should feel like a gentle pulling motion—use caution not to physically pull too hard and stress your hamstring. The purpose of the drill is to tune in to the mechanics of your pedal stroke, making each part powerful.

_ *Find the zone (or find the edge):* Start on what feels like light tension on a flat road. If you were biking outside, it feels like enough tension to create the friction between your tire and the road, but it's easy and smooth. Start at around 80 rpms. Gradually add tension every 30-60 seconds, a little bit at a time, trying to keep yourself at 80 rpms. The challenge on this drill is that you are trying to keep the same cadence with quiet, smooth pedal strokes even as you are adding tension. Keep adding tension until you feel like you've found your "edge:" it is tough to maintain, but you haven't lost good form yet. Hold for another 30 seconds before taking off the tension for a recovery period. You can try this drill again at 90 rpms, and at 100 rpms.

_ *Attack and breakaway:* This is designed to simulate a cyclist overtaking and passing another cyclist in a race situation. In a seated position, adjust tension so you feel like you're on a flat road or a slight hill. Start at around 80 rpms—it should feel easy. Hold for 30-60 seconds, then accelerate to 100 rpms. Hold for another 30-60 seconds. Then quickly to accelerate to 110 rpms, simulating passing someone. Hold for 30 seconds. Decelerate slightly back to 100 rpms and hold for 60 seconds. This mimics the fast pace needed to maintain a pass, and then hold the lead over another cyclist. Always maintain good form. Once you get the hang of it, try this at a harder tension to simulate passing on a hill.

- *Spin-ups:* At a moderate tension in a seated position, start at 80 rpms. Take 5 seconds to accelerate up to 110 rpms: hold this for 20 seconds, then take another 5 seconds to decelerate. Recover at an easy pace for 20 seconds. Repeat. Try this on repeats for 2-3 minutes. The goal of this drill is to practice high speeds with smooth form and powerful pedal strokes.

These are just a few drills to get you started. Drills are a fabulous way to build stamina, mental toughness, and correct technique. They are a fun way to give variety to any cycle workout.

Bike Shorts: Chapter 9

Stretches

After a cool-down of pedaling at an easy pace for about 5 minutes, the instructor will have you stretch. Here are a few key stretches that will help assist in recovery and promote muscle health. Be sure to stretch after each workout and again later in the day if you feel sore or stiff. Here are a few stretches you should do after a cycle class.

Hamstring: This group of muscles is located in the upper back part of your leg. Start standing straight with flat back. Place one leg forward with knee straight and heel touching the floor in a staggered stance. Now raise your hands above your head and slowly hinge forward at the hip, lowering your upper half to about a 45° angle. Feel the stretch in the back of your leg. Hold for 15-60 seconds. Switch legs and repeat.

Hip flexors: These muscles are on the front of your body near your groin, where your legs connect to your pelvis/hip area. Stagger your stance so you are in a lunge position with right leg in front. Keeping your top half upright, reach your left arm up while slowly lowering deeper into the lunge. Breathe into the stretch as you feel it lengthening and releasing tension. Switch sides and repeat.

Piriformis/Gluteal: These muscles are located in your buttock area. While seated on a mat, bend your knees. Cross one leg over the other and rest your ankle just below your knee on top of your thigh. Bring your legs into your chest to deepen the stretch. Uncross your legs and repeat on the opposite side.

Quadriceps: This is a group of muscles on top of your thighs. While standing, bend one knee, bringing your heel toward your buttocks. Grasp the top of your foot (where your shoelaces are) and hold your foot close to your body, feeling the stretch in the front part of your thigh. Hold and breathe into the stretch. Repeat on the opposite side.

It's also a good idea to stretch your arms up overhead, opening up your chest and relaxing your shoulder blades down. Do a few shoulder rolls and move your chin side to side to release any tension in your neck. Breathe slowly and deeply throughout your stretching, thinking about releasing tension and lengthening muscles.

Keep reading for information on proper nutrition for before, during and after a cycle class.

Bike Shorts: Chapter 10

Nutrition and hydration for cycling

Nutrition is an important part of a healthy lifestyle. Coupled with exercise, good nutrition can help maintain or lose weight, prevent and/or treat chronic disease, and help promote healthy immunity, improved mental state, and a myriad of other benefits.

First, it's good to know what are good food sources of carbohydrates and protein.

Good sources of carbohydrate include:
  _ Grains: bread, pasta, rice, cereal, crackers, etc.
  _ Milk and yogurt
  _ Fruit and fruit juices
  _ Starchy vegetables, such as potatoes, yams, peas, corn, and squash
  _ Beans and lentils (legumes)

Note: other sources of carbohydrate are sweets and desserts. These should be enjoyed only occasionally.

Good sources of protein include:
  _ Meat, fish, and poultry
  _ Eggs
  _ Dairy products (cheese, yogurt, milk)
  _ Beans and lentils (legumes)
  _ Nuts and seeds
  _ Soybeans and soybean products (like tofu)

There are some specific things you'll want to tweak in your diet to optimize your workout and recovery.

Before exercise: If you do an early morning cycle class, I'm impressed!

There are a couple of nutrition considerations with early morning workouts. If your goal is to train your body to burn fat more efficiently, there is no need to eat before exercising. There's some great research that shows that working out in a semi-fasted or fasted state (such as when you wake up and haven't eaten since dinner last night) can train your body to oxidize fat more efficiently. This means you burn fat more easily, rather than relying on carbohydrate stores or dietary carbohydrate (food you just ate).[2]

However, there is a drawback to this method. While you can train your body to burn fat, which is helpful for endurance athletes, your workout intensity and quality will be compromised. This is because, for a really hard sprint or intense work, your body uses carbohydrate. If this is unavailable (because you haven't eaten yet), you won't be able to work as hard. Or, if you are drawing on carbohydrate stores in your body (in the form of a storage sugar in your muscles and liver called glycogen), they can be depleted quickly. This means that when you sprint or do intense work, it will feel much harder and more fatiguing than it would have if you had eaten some carbohydrate.

If you feel weak, faint, dizzy, or easily fatigued during your cycle class, be sure to eat something beforehand. Here are some ideas:

If it is 2-4 hours before a workout:
- Oatmeal with berries and milk
- Whole grain toast, almond butter, and apple slices

- Eggs, whole grain mini-bagel, orange juice
- Brown rice bowl with chicken and veggies
- Berry, spinach, and yogurt smoothie

If it is 30-60 minutes before a workout, you need to eat foods that are easily digestible and low in fiber. This will allow the food to be metabolized more quickly in your body, allowing it to be available for fuel during a cycle class. It will also minimize any gastrointestinal distress, such as diarrhea, gas, bloating, or cramping. Try these ideas:

- White mini-bagel
- Pretzels
- Rice cakes
- Fruit juice
- Sports drink such as Gatorade
- Sports gummies, chews, or gels

During a workout: You don't necessarily need to eat before a workout if the cycle class is going to be around 60 minutes or less. If you usually feel fine during exercise without specifically eating *for* the exercise, you don't need to purposefully eat. For anything longer than 90 minutes, be sure to fuel before and/or during your workout. Eating a simple carbohydrate that is easily digested is a smart move for workouts longer than 90 minutes.

You would need about 30-60 grams of carbohydrate per hour.[3] It looks like this:

- About 16 oz Gatorade
- 2 packets of Gu
- Sports gummies or chews (check the label for grams of carbohydrate)
- 2 oz pretzels
- 2 tablespoons honey
- A roll with jam

Keep in mind that you only need to eat if it is a really long ride, over 90 minutes, or if you feel weak or easily fatigued, like you are running out of fuel. If you have breakthrough hunger during a cycle class, that's a great sign that you need to eat something prior to your cycle class.

After a workout: When your class is done and you've worked up a good sweat, this is the perfect opportunity to recover and refuel. Some amazing things happen in your body after a workout. Certain hormones in your body get to work, remodeling and rebuilding bone and muscle tissue. That storage sugar, called glycogen, can get restored if you feed your body correctly. It goes into the muscle and liver, ready and waiting to fuel your next workout.

There's something called a "metabolic window" of time after exercise where your body is ready and willing to absorb nutrients and repair itself. Researchers are in debate about how long exactly this metabolic window is, and, truthfully, it likely varies between people and circumstances. It's been shown to be anywhere from 30 minutes to 48 hours after a workout that the body is rebuilding and repairing.

No matter what time the window "closes," certainly immediately after working out you'll want to eat something to help this process along. Within about 60 minutes, be sure to eat a meal, or at least a snack. Something with both a carbohydrate and a protein are crucial. Here are some ideas:

- Chocolate milk
- A fruit and yogurt smoothie
- Burrito with meat or beans, rice, and veggies
- A turkey sandwich with veggies and cheese
- Quinoa bowl with black beans, cheese, avocado, and peppers
- Sandwich with whole grain bread, almond butter, and jam

There are some other interesting and promising foods that can help with recovery. Beet root juice, tart cherry juice, pomegranate, and blueberries likely all have benefits.[4]

Protein is key to help build and repair muscle. Try to eat about 20 grams of protein within about 60-90 minutes after your cycle class. Milk is especially good at helping with muscle recovery. It has an amino acid called leucine that has been shown to be very effective at building and rebuilding muscle tissue. Here are some ideas to get your protein intake, with vegan options at the bottom of the list:

- 2 oz cheese
- 2 eggs
- 16 oz milk or chocolate milk
- 8 oz yogurt
- 3 oz meat, fish, or chicken
- 2 c cereal with 1 c milk
- 2 oz nuts
- 2 c bean soup or lentil chili

Aside from eating before, during, and after workouts, eating an overall healthy and balanced diet can help you with your fitness and wellness goals. This means including a base of plenty of fruits, vegetables, whole grains, legumes, nuts and seeds. Include lean proteins such as lean chicken, pork, and beef. Fish, dairy products, eggs, and tofu are great sources of protein as well. In addition, healthy fats are a crucial part of a healthy diet. These come from foods like avocado, olives and olive oil, almonds and walnuts, and salmon. Eating a variety of foods allows for adequate nutrient intake.

Hydration: For a 30 to 60-minute cycle class, drinking sips of water throughout the class (when you are thirsty) is likely going to provide you with adequate hydration. If you are cycling for longer than 90 minutes, use Gatorade or another sports drink to provide needed carbohydrate and electrolytes for your ride.

If it is particularly hot or humid, you may need more fluids than usual. Drink according to your needs for that ride and the environmental conditions. If your urine is light yellow after working out, you drank enough. If it is dark or concentrated, drink more.

Measuring sweat rate may be useful if you regularly ride longer than 90 minutes. This is a way to measure how much you sweat in a workout session. If you know how much you sweat, you can know how much to drink to replace that sweat (fluid loss). Ideally, you'll want to prevent a fluid loss of more than 2% of your body weight to prevent dehydration and decreased performance.[5] It takes a bit of math, but stay with me. It'll pay off. Here's how you do it:

1. Empty your bladder. Weigh yourself before you exercise with as little clothing as possible.
2. Exercise until you sweat! Keep track of how many ounces you drink. Complete your workout.
3. Weigh yourself again in the same amount of clothing. See how much weight you lost.
4. Use these steps to determine how much weight you lost from sweat:

    -   Starting weight–ending weight=weight you lost during the workout.

    -   Convert your weight loss into ounces. 1 pound = 16 ounces.

    -   Add what you drank to your fluid loss.
    -   This is the grand total of your sweat loss.

Lost? It makes more sense with the numbers plugged in. It looks like this: Let's say you weighed 160 pounds after urinating and before exercising, and you drank 16 ounces while exercising. After you were done, you weighed 158 pounds. That means you lost two pounds! You also drank a pound of fluid (16 ounces) while you were exercising. What if you hadn't drunk that 16 ounces? You would have lost three pounds instead of two. This means you lost three pounds of pure sweat while you worked out. Time to replace that fluid by drinking! Drink 16 ounces for every pound lost. That means you need to drink 32 ounces in this case, because you lost two pounds---each pound is 16 ounces, so 16 x 2 = 32 ounces---over the next few hours. Next time, you will know that you usually sweat about 3 pounds of fluid loss over the course of your workout. So you can drink throughout your workout to replace that sweat loss.

Here's what it looks like as a formula:
Starting weight 160 pounds
Ending weight 158 pounds
Drank 16 ounces while exercising
160–158=2 pounds lost while exercising
2 pounds lost + 16 ounces (1 pound) drank = 3 pounds of total sweat loss that occurred.

Still confused? Just Google the term "sweat rate calculator" and a number of options will come up. You don't have to think—you just plug in the numbers. Data.gssiweb.com has an excellent one. Easy!

Bike Shorts: Chapter 11

Sample workouts

Ok, so you've read the book. You are totally convinced that not only will you look dang good in bike shorts, but you are going to rock your ride!

Music is key to feeling motivated. A good playlist can help keep you going, and a strong beat or chorus helps push through the intense parts. If you are looking for good music ideas, check out websites like rockmyrun.com, workoutmusic.com, or the "Fitness & Workout" genre in the iTunes store.

When you've compiled your playlist, try it with these sample workouts to get you started. Or just go to an indoor cycle class, where the instructor has done all the prep work for you!

Workout 1: Hills and drills

	Time	Heart rate zone	RPE
Warm up	5-10 minutes	50-65%	2-4
Hill — moderate tension, seated push	1 minute moderate tension, 1 minute harder, 1 minute hardest	65-75%	5-8
Push/pull	5 minutes	65-75%	4-8

drill			
Hill — heavy tension, out of saddle	3 minute continuous hill	75-85%	4-9
Spin ups drill	3 minutes total	75-95% during sprint portion	8-10 for sprint portion
Switchback hill — climb moderate hill, but every 45 seconds add tension for a steep "switchback" around a "bend" in the road for 10-20 pedal strokes	5 minutes alternating between moderate hill and heavy "switchbacks"	65-85%	6-9
Find the zone drill	5 minutes	65-85%	6-9
Cool down	5-10 minutes	50-65%	2-4

Workout 2: Endurance circuit

	Time	Heart rate zone	RPE
Warm up	5-10 minutes	50-65%	2-4
Seated flat	3 minutes	65-75%	4-6
Standing flat	3 minutes	65-75%	4-6
Seated hill	3 minutes	65-75%	4-6
Standing hill	3 minutes	65-75%	4-6
Jumps (every 8 counts up and down)	3 minutes	65-75%	4-6
Repeat: Seated flat	3 minutes	65-75%	4-6
Standing flat	3 minutes	65-75%	4-6
Seated hill	3 minutes	65-75%	4-6
Standing hill	3 minutes	65-75%	4-6
Jumps	3 minutes	65-75%	4-6
Cool down	5-10 minutes	50%	2-4

Workout 3: Speed work

	Time	Heart Rate Zone	RPE
Warm up	5-10 minutes	50%	2-4
Seated flat, 90-100 rpms	3 minutes	65-75%	4-6
Recover 70-80 rpms	1 minute	50%	2-4
Sprint, seated flat, 110 rpms	30 seconds	85-95%	7-10
Recover 70-80 rpms	1 minute	50%	2-4
Standing flat, 70 rpms	3 minutes	65-75%	4-6
Recover 70-80 rpms	1 minute	50%	2-4
Sprint, seated flat, 110 rpms	30 seconds	85-95%	7-10
Recover 70-80 rpms	1 minute	50%	2-4
Attack and breakaway drill	1-5 minutes	75-95%	5-10
Cool down	5-10 minutes	50%	2-4

Bike Shorts: Conclusion

Indoor cycling can be a fun addition to an active lifestyle, or it can be a first step on the way to health and wellness. Seasoned cyclists love the options it gives for winter training and specific interval work. Newbies love the safe and effective workout it offers within a group setting.

Regardless of your age or fitness level, indoor cycling can be a valuable addition to your routine. Use this guidebook to help you hone your skills and achieve a higher fitness level.

If you liked the book, please leave a positive review on Amazon. Thanks for reading, and happy riding!

Biker Shorts: References

1) Warburton, D.E.R, Nicol, C.W., & Bredin, S.S.D. (2006). Heath benefits of physical activity: the evidence. *Canadian Medical Association Journal,* 174(6): 801-809.

2) Burke, L.M. (2015). Re-examining high-fat diets for sports performance: did we call the 'nail in the coffin' too soon? *Sports Medicine,* 45 (suppl 1):S33-S49.

3) Burke, L.M., Hawley, J.A., Wong, S.H.S., & Jeukendrup, A.E. (2011). Carbohydrates for training and competition. *Journal of Sport Sciences,* 29(S1): S17-S27.

4) Sousa, M., Teixeira, V.H, & Soares, J. (2014). Dietary strategies to recover from exercise-induced muscle damage. *International Journal of Food Sciences and Nutrition,* 65(2): 151-163.

5) Position stand: exercise and fluid replacement. (2007). *Medicine & Science in Sports & Exercise,* 39, 377-390.

6) Castronovo, A.M., Conforto, S., Schmid, M., Bibbo, D., & D'Alessio, T. (2013). How to assess performance in cycling: the multivariate nature of influencing factors and related indicators. *Frontiers in Physiology,* 4:116.

7) Stebbins, C.L., Moore, J.L., & Casazza, G. (2014). Effects of cadence on aerobic capacity following a prolonged, varied intensity cycling trial. *Journal of Sports Science and Medicine,* 13, 114-119.

Made in the USA
San Bernardino, CA
20 February 2017